THE
RESISTANCEBAND
WORKOUT

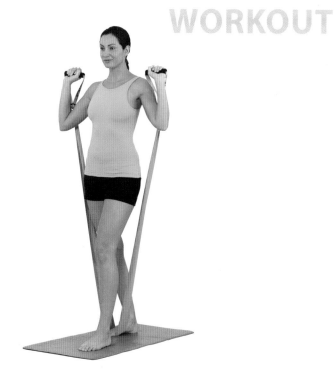

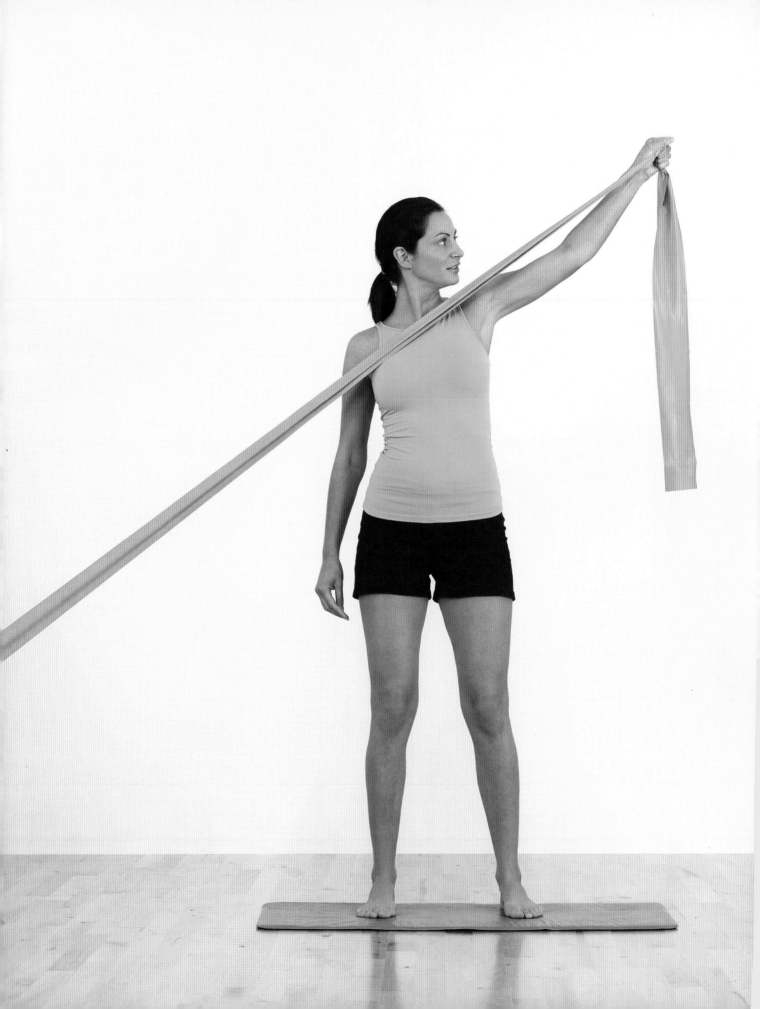

THE RESISTANCE BAND WORKOUT

John Edward Kennett

p

This is a Parragon Publishing Book
First published in 2006

Parragon Publishing
Queen Street House
4 Queen Street
Bath BA1 1HE, UK

ISBN: 1-40548-953-7
Printed in China

Created and produced by the Bridgewater Book Company Ltd
Photography: Ian Parsons
Hair and make-up stylist: Johan van der Merwe
Models: Katie Lawrie and Kevin Dixon
Illustrations: John Woodcock

The publisher would like to thank the following for permission to
reproduce copyright material: Brooke Fasani/Corbis (page 6) and
Ben Welsh/zefa/Corbis (page 7).

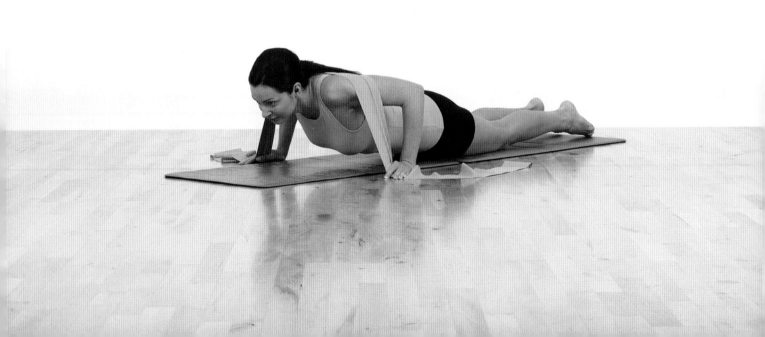

contents

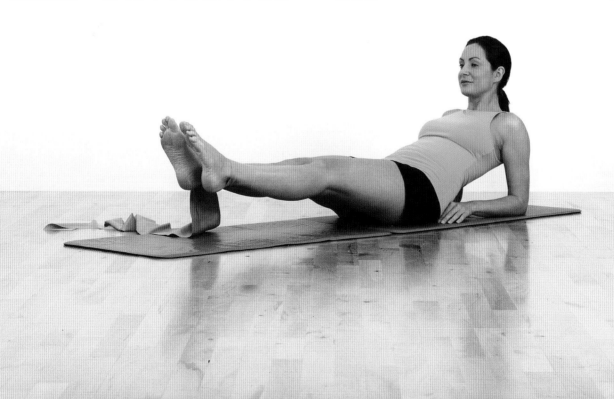

Resistance bands are amazing fitness tools. Their ability to improve your fitness and your strength, develop your muscle speed and stamina, and increase your body's mobility seems almost too good to be true for such simple objects, and until recently they were seldom used by anyone other than top sports people. However, now resistance bands are starting to get the attention that they deserve, and with this book you will discover everything you need to know about using them.

With the assistance of this book you can build strength, speed, and muscle stamina, decrease body fat, improve your flexibility and balance, and exercise and strengthen specific muscles that machines would miss. You can achieve your goal with a combination of resistance band exercises and a positive attitude that motivates you to keep up a consistent program. You can exercise just about anywhere, it does not depend on the weather, and it is inexpensive. With this insightful book, the resistance band is no longer a secret.

Many people want to get fit, and take up a sport—tennis, golf, soccer, cycling, swimming, skiing—in order to become fit. In doing so, though, they may soon suffer injuries that prevent them from pursuing the enjoyment of sport and the fundamental physiological and psychological health benefits that fitness gives them. So remember, it is not about playing a sport to become fit—it is about becoming fit in order to play and enjoy sport.

Research proves that resistance band training provides as much benefit in fitness and strength gains as those achieved on cumbersome and expensive weight-training equipment. The reason is simple—as the elastic band is stretched, so resistance increases, providing progressive stimulus to your muscles.

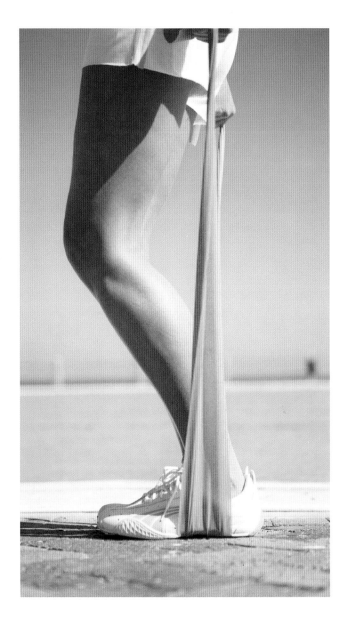

introduction

This book will guide you through some of the fundamental principles of exercise, teaching you how to prepare your body and motivate your mind to ensure you attain and maintain your desired results using resistance bands. You will gain an insight into how specific body types react to different resistance band exercises. You will learn that stretching is not warming up and warming up is not stretching, as well as the importance of a warm-down after you have exercised. You will be able to determine the correct percentage of your maximum heart rate within which to exercise, enabling you to lose body fat, increase your fitness, build muscle strength, or a combination of all three. This will enable you to choose and combine the resistance band exercises into a routine best suited to your body type and your desired outcome.

Until recently, resistance bands were mostly used in remedial physiotherapy, enabling patients to recover range of motion, strength, and stability after injury. Knowledge of sports science has grown over recent years, and top sports people now utilize resistance band training to improve their performance. If you work with the resistance band, you can gain advantages in your fitness exercise regime and chosen sport.

CAUTION

Consult your health advisor before embarking on any new fitness program, especially if you suffer from or have a history of high blood pressure or heart conditions.

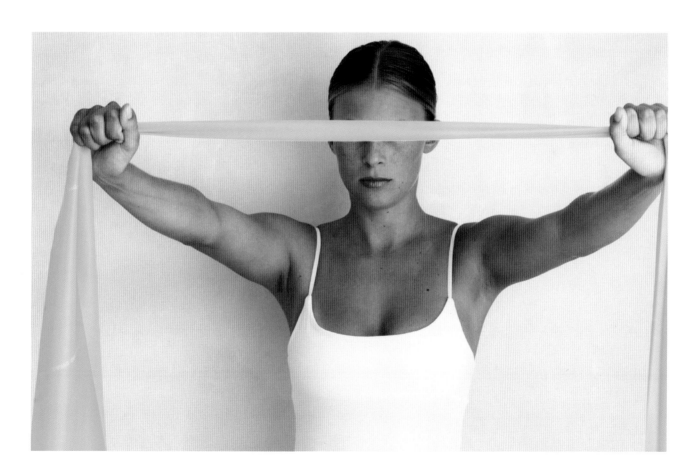

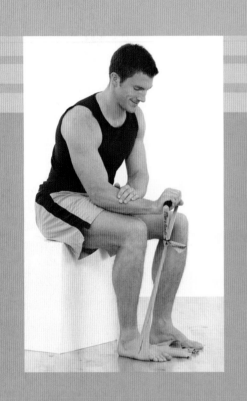
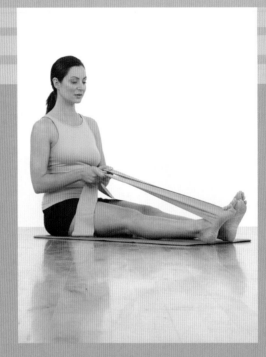
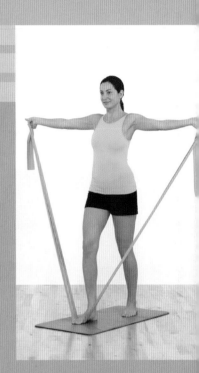

1
resistance band

Resistance band training offers you a number of benefits, and in this chapter you will learn how and why resistance bands work simply and effectively. You will discover the fundamental principles of exercise as practiced by top sports people and dancers. Exercising within a specific heart-rate range, with an understanding of how body type enters into the equation, will empower you to decide which type of resistance band exercise suits your needs. You will also learn how to maintain your exercise program and enjoy the thrill of knowing that resistance band exercises can change your body, motivating you to reach your desired goal.

From beginners to seasoned athletes, we can all benefit by adding resistance bands and resistance tubes to our training programs. There are many elastic band resistance products on the market, most developed from the two basic options of the resistance band and the resistance tube. Neither differs from the other in principle, concept, or mechanics. In general, all the exercises can be done with either bands or tubing, depending upon your preference, and, unless specified, the use of the resistance band is identical to the resistance tube.

Resistance band training is simple: the more the elastic band is stretched, the more the resistance increases, and likewise, the band will contract as the force decreases. Neither type of elastic resistance relies on gravity, unlike most exercise machines and the classic free weights such as the dumbbell; instead, resistance is dependent upon how far the resistance band is stretched, and continuously and increasingly places demands on your muscles as they contract throughout the whole range of motion.

Both bands and tubing come in different lengths and many resistance levels. The bands or tubes are color-coded according to their resistance levels. Different manufacturers use different color schemes for their bands and tubes, but generally both the color and resistance of the band or tube start light and progress through to darker colors, which represent increased resistance.

The possibilities of resistance bands are limited only by your imagination. They let you move more freely and achieve a greater range of motion than machines, which control where you start and stop. This enables you to create resistance from any direction—high overhead, below from floor level,

or to the side, for example. By adjusting your angle of movement, moving the fixed point higher or lower, several exercises can be combined. Resistance bands let you imitate movements that you do in real life, and exercise muscles that machines miss. Many different exercises can be performed with a single resistance band.

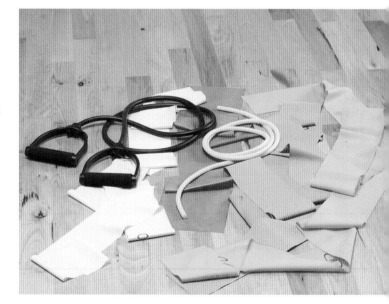

how resistance bands work

Resistance band exercising will assist in strengthening the muscles involved in respiration, facilitating the flow of air in and out of your lungs; aid in strengthening the heart, to improve its pumping efficiency and reduce your resting heart rate; tone the muscles throughout your body, which can improve your overall circulation and reduce blood pressure; and increase the number of red blood cells in your body, improving oxygen transportation.

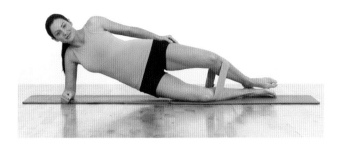

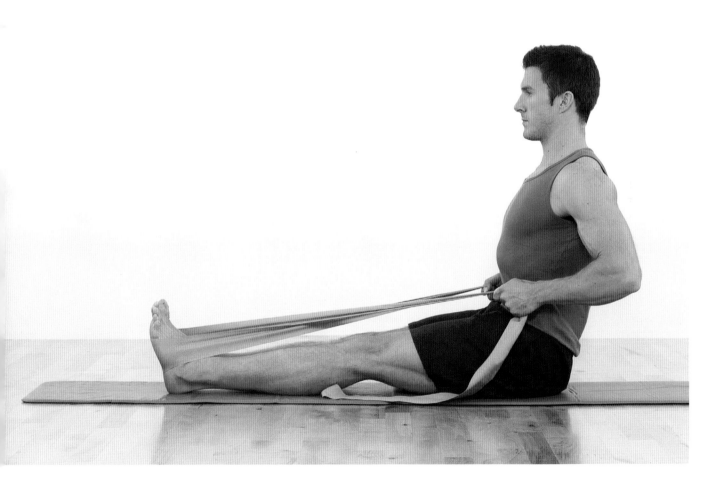

When working with resistance bands, it is extremely useful to have an understanding of basic anatomy. This makes it much easier to appreciate the many positive effects that training with resistance bands can have on different parts of the body.

Muscles and bones are collectively called the musculoskeletal system. Bones give structural and postural support to the body in conjunction with the muscles' ability to contract, enabling movement. The mechanical stresses imposed by resistance band exercises can improve bone condition. It has been shown in studies that where these stresses are applied on the skeleton the most, more mineral salts are deposited and more collagen fibers are produced, causing both the density and also the size of the bone to increase.

Bones are linked together via joints, which can be fixed, slightly movable, or free:

• Fixed, or fibrous, joints, such as the suture type found in the skull, bind the bones tightly together with fibrous connective tissue, permitting no movement between them.

• Slightly movable, or cartilaginous, joints, such as the pads of cartilage found in between the vertebrae of the spine, move by compression of the cartilage.

• Freely movable, or synovial, joints are of five different types:

1 Ball and socket joints, such as the hip and shoulder joints, are the most movable of all joints, enabling movement of limbs in many different directions.

2 Hinge joints, such as the knee and elbow, move in one directional plane only.

3 Gliding joints, such as the carpal bones in the hand and the tarsal bones in the foot, enable the bones to glide against each other and are the least movable of this type.

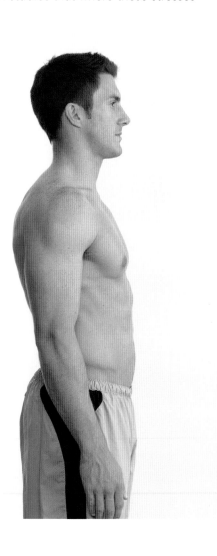

basic anatomy

4 Pivot joints enable a rotary movement about one axis, such as the first two cervical vertebrae, the atlas and axis, which let the head rotate.

5 Saddle joints are found only in the thumbs and provide movement about two axes, similar to a ball and socket joint, enabling the thumb to oppose the index finger.

Bones, tendons, and ligaments are not able to make your body move—only muscles can do this. Varying in size and in shape, there are three types of muscle tissue which have different purposes:

• Involuntary muscles, known as smooth muscles, differ from other muscle types in structure and function. Smooth muscles are found within the "walls" of hollow organs such as blood vessels and the bladder, and work automatically. Regular exercise with a resistance band can develop this muscle type, improving the muscles' efficiency.

• Cardiac muscle exists only in the heart. It is myogenic, meaning that it stimulates its own contraction without a requisite electrical impulse. The resistance band exercises and workout routines will effectively exercise your heart, enabling it to work more efficiently.

• Skeletal muscles, or voluntary muscles, are generally consciously controlled. Composed of a group of specialized strands of elastic tissues, bound together in bundles and contained in a sheath called fasculi, they combine to form the muscle belly. The ends of these bundles extend to form a tendon that attaches to other parts of the body; usually one end, the head or origin, is attached to a relatively stationary bone; the other end, the insertion, is attached across a joint to another bone. Muscles with two heads are known as the biceps, three heads as

the triceps, and four as the quadriceps. Working out with a resistance band can strengthen, lengthen, and improve both your muscles' endurance and flexibility.

Skeletal muscles contain two types of muscle fibers. Type I "slow twitch" fibers are good for endurance and are slow to tire. High repetition, low intensity resistance band exercise will stimulate and increase the proliferation of these fibers. Type II "fast twitch" fibers are divided into type IIa for great strength, lasting over modest periods, and type IIb, also used for short bursts of speed and power but tiring even faster. Low repetition, high intensity resistance band exercise will build "fast twitch" muscle fibers.

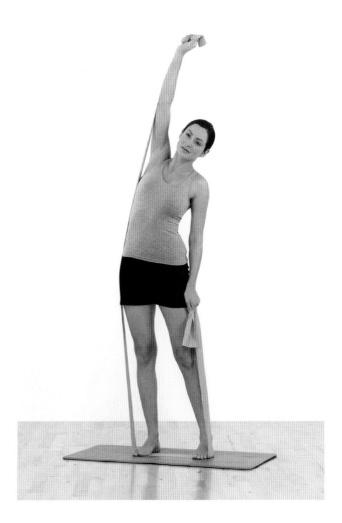

The muscles

For a muscle to contract, it needs large amounts of energy and a message to be sent from the brain to initiate its movement. The body's energy is provided by a compound called adenosine triphosphate (ATP), which is made in muscle cells. Muscles have a store of energy generating ATP for about 10 seconds of exercise before depleting. The muscle will then convert ATP from carbohydrate that is stored in the form of glycogen. Waste products are created, such as lactic acid, which the body removes from the muscles to prevent buildup.

Each muscle fiber is innervated by a nerve called a motor neuron. A single motor neuron supplies many muscle fibers and is known as a motor unit. The nervous and muscular systems communicate via the neuromuscular junction. Here the muscle fiber is triggered by a nerve impulse that bridges the gap between the muscle fiber and nerve ending. This happens indirectly by the secretion of a neurotransmitter called acetylcholine. Depending upon the muscle, a single motor neuron can innervate from one to many hundreds of muscle fibers.

All the body's movements involve the action of more than one muscle. The muscle primarily responsible for movement becomes known as the agonist. As it contracts, the opposing muscle, called the antagonist, relaxes to enable movement. For example, when flexing the elbow, the biceps brachii muscle acts as the agonist by contracting. The triceps brachii is the antagonist. The antagonist can also contract at the same time as the agonist, to control or slow down a movement.

By becoming familiar with the muscles that make up your body, you will become more familiar with the muscles that you are working, making it easier to feel and visualize which exercises are helping you to make the improvements you desire.

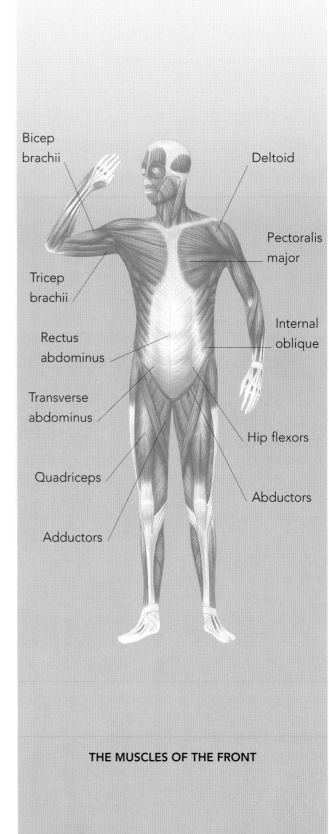

Bicep brachii

Deltoid

Pectoralis major

Tricep brachii

Internal oblique

Rectus abdominus

Transverse abdominus

Hip flexors

Quadriceps

Abductors

Adductors

THE MUSCLES OF THE FRONT

Shoulders, arms, chest, and upper back

Strengthening the shoulders, arms, chest, and upper back improves functions such as carrying, lifting objects, lifting overhead, pushing, and pulling. Sport-specific training of the shoulders and arms benefits sports such as tennis, cricket, volleyball, and swimming, as well as the martial arts. Balancing overworked chest muscles with upper back muscles will help to maintain a good posture, prevent injury, and assist with rehabilitation after injury.

Abdominals and lower back

The abdominal and lower back muscles are collectively known as the "core." "Core stability" is the ability to control the position and movement of the central portion of the body. Strengthening the abdominal and lower back muscles helps to reduce the risk of injury from bad posture and improves the foundation for all arm and leg movements. In addition, strengthening the abdominals and lower back can prevent and improve lower back pain.

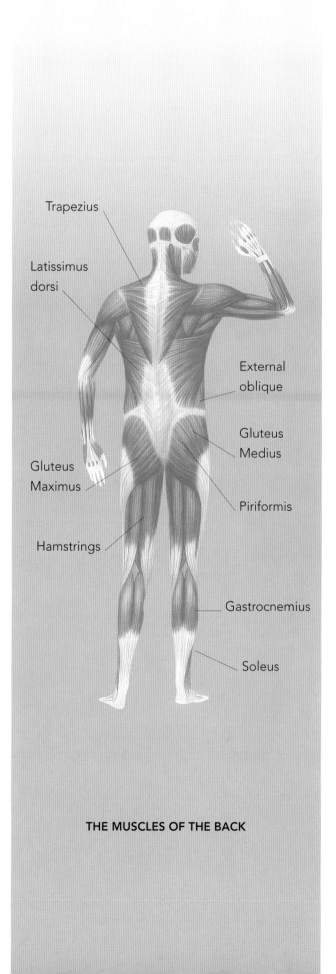

Trapezius

Latissimus dorsi

External oblique

Gluteus Medius

Gluteus Maximus

Piriformis

Hamstrings

Gastrocnemius

Soleus

THE MUSCLES OF THE BACK

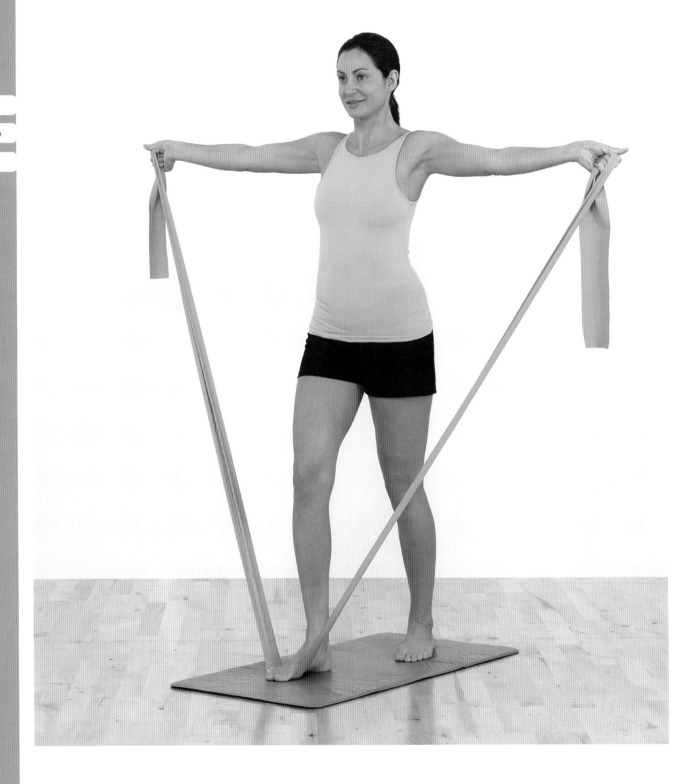

Hips, thighs, lower legs, and ankles

The hip and thigh regions are one of the most important areas you can strengthen. Connecting the legs to the trunk, the hips provide a stable base for the "core."

The hips are fundamental in transferring your center of gravity during walking and running. The gluteal muscles provide pelvic stability. Weakness of the gluteal muscles is linked to back pain, knee pain, hip pain, and repetitive ankle injuries. Also, imbalances of strength and flexibility between your quadriceps and hamstrings can be linked to knee pain.

The lower leg muscles and ankles are important for stability, for locomotion, and for action within the walking and running cycle, known as gait. Improving your lower leg strength can go a long way toward improving your balance and stability, especially when participating in sports that require quick changes of direction, such as soccer, tennis, and basketball.

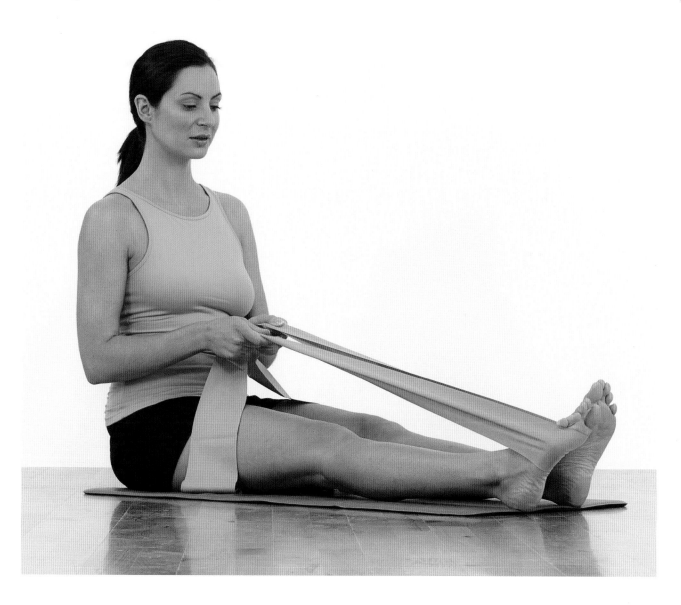

The way our bodies look and respond to different types of exercise is basically determined by our genetics. Other factors include how active you were while growing up, your diet during your childhood and teenage years, and your current diet and activity levels.

Often people become disheartened when exercising to lose weight, as they unexpectedly find that their size "increases." The reason is that an increase in muscle bulk within an area with noticeably high body fat can initially cause an increase in that area's overall size. This occurs because anaerobic exercise tends to cause muscles to bulk and increase in size more than aerobic exercise does, and because the body fat has not yet decreased sufficiently and is overlying any area of increased muscle bulk. This can be avoided by exercising correctly for your body type. Body type does not describe how much fat or muscle your body has. It simply means where on your body it would be evident if weight was being added or lost.

X-types

X-types have the classic hourglass-shaped body, which proportionally tends to add mass to both the upper and lower parts of the body quite easily, while the waist will be more slender. They will also lose mass proportionally from the upper and lower bodies.

Aerobic weight-management resistance band exercises for both upper and lower bodies will benefit the X-type. As they slim down, the exercise can turn more anaerobic.

Y-types

Y-types are bigger on the top half of their body, with a tendency to bulk up from the waist up. Y-types carry weight and mass in their upper back and chest, and their arms are usually large as well.

To reduce the size of the upper part of your body, use an aerobic exercise weight-management plan on

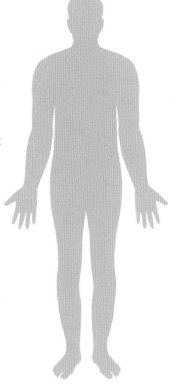

X

Y

body types

your upper body, with a low intensity of resistance band and high repetitions. Y-types will benefit from moderate to high intensity anaerobic resistance band exercises to the lower half of the body.

If you are overweight, reduce the resistance on the upper body, because fat will be pushed outward as muscle is built.

I-types

I-types carry the same proportion of weight on the upper body as on the lower, are not tapered in their midsection, and do not have many curves.

Provided I-types are not overweight, they can perform both anaerobic and aerobic resistance band exercises. If you are overweight, however, use predominantly aerobic weight-management resistance band exercises.

A-types

A-types are the classic pear shape. Their upper bodies may not be small, yet they are still considerably smaller than their lower half. A-types tend to put on weight or mass in their thighs, hips, behind the knees, and even in the calves and ankles.

A-types should use a low-intensity weight-management resistance band exercises at high repetitions for the lower body. You can use anaerobic resistance band exercises of moderate to high resistance at low repetitions for your upper body. If you are overweight, resistance should not be too high for the upper body, because fat will be pushed outward as muscle is built.

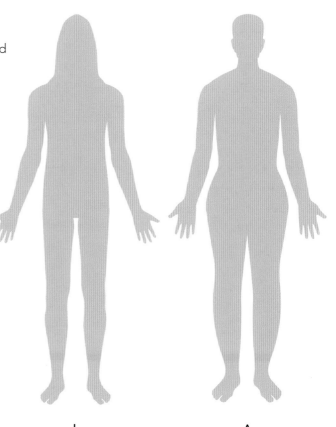

I   A

AEROBIC AND ANAEROBIC EXERCISE

Aerobic exercise, such as gentle jogging, is replicated by moderate to low levels of resistance band intensity with high repetitions, maintaining an increased heart rate, but not entering into the anaerobic zone. The aerobic exercise zone is also known as the weight management zone. Anaerobic exercise uses muscles in a brief, high intensity activity where oxygen requirements cannot meet the demand of the activity, increasing the breathing and heart rate very quickly—for example, when you are sprinting. A high tension resistance band enabling only low repetitions before fatigue will add to muscle bulk.

To ensure you get the maximum benefit from resistance band exercises, and indeed any exercise, check your heart rate during your fitness session. The number of heartbeats per minute is one of the easiest measures to take, and as you become fitter you will be able to increase your heart rate without straining your heart.

Your target heart rate (THR) is the recommended number of heartbeats per minute for your age and fitness level while exercising. It is derived as a percentage of your maximum heart rate. It is important to remain within the target heart zone to ensure you are exercising with the correct intensity. If you are exercising above your THR, you are exercising too vigorously; below your THR, and you are not exercising with enough vigor.

To take your own pulse, place your two forefingers on your carotid arteries, found either side of your neck, just below the angle of the jaw, between the neck muscle and windpipe. Do not use your thumb because it has a pulse of its own.

Time your heartbeat for 15 seconds. Multiply the number of beats over 15 seconds by four. This will give you your beats per minute.

ZONE LIMIT

Zone	Target heart rate %	ratio of calories burned (fat/other calories)	Benefit
Warm-up	50–60	85/15	Warm-up and warm-down zones. Decreases body fat, blood pressure, and cholesterol.
Weight management	60–70	85/15	As above, but burns more total calories.
Aerobic	70–80	50/50	Improves your cardiovascular and respiratory system, and increases the size and strength of your heart. Builds more "slow twitch" muscle fibers.
Anaerobic	80–90	15/85	High-intensity zone, burning more calories, improving the cardiorespiratory system, and increasing endurance. Builds more "fast twitch" muscle fibers.

target heart rate

Example

20 beats in 15 seconds = 80 beats per minute

Your maximum heart rate is your age subtracted from 220 for men, and your age subtracted from 226 for women. This number, your maximum heart rate of beats per minute, should not be exceeded during any physical activity.

Example

A 40-year-old man has a maximum heart rate of 180 beats per minute (220 – 40 = 180).

From this, you can then work out the upper and lower limits for your heart rate in the different zones. Simply multiply your maximum heart rate by the upper and lower target heart rates listed in the table opposite.

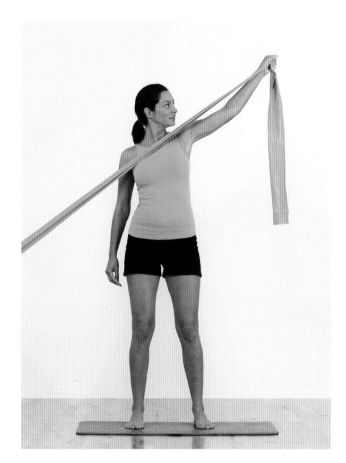

HEART RATE CALCULATIONS

Maximum heart rate for women = 226 - age

Maximum heart rate for men = 220 - age

Upper target heart rate =
(Maximum heart rate) x (upper % of zone)

Lower target heart rate =
(Maximum heart rate) x (lower % of zone)

Example

For a 28-year-old woman who wishes to exercise in the aerobic zone:

Maximum heart rate: 226 – 28 = 198

Upper heart rate: 198 x 0.8 = 158

Lower heart rate: 198 x 0.7 = 139

Thus, a 28-year-old woman exercising in the aerobic zone would maintain their target heart rate between 139 and 158 beats per minute.

To get the pulse count range, simply divide by 4, giving 35 to 39 beats over 15 seconds.

Think of a time in the past when you had a peak moment when you felt good, fit, strong and able, energized, and excited—it could be a sporting moment, or even after being able to climb a steep flight of stairs or a challenging hill. Please take a moment, now, and reflect on that time and relive it in your mind. Where were you, what were you doing? Feel as many of the sensory elements of that time as you can recall and bring it to life again—recreate that time as if you were there now and feel alive again.

Now project your thoughts forward in time, to your reason for exercising with resistance bands and to your desired state. Notice the increased fitness, strength, and mobility you can gain. See yourself in that moment, and the benefits you have gained—energy to tackle stairs with ease, improved balance, more vigor to play with your children, greater potential in your sport, or whatever is the desired outcome of these exercises. Notice, too, the improvements to your lifestyle, such as the reduction in stress and the joy that brings you, and hear people telling you how good you look, and asking you how you achieved it.

Motivation is a force that makes us "do," turning desires and goals into action. There are two types of motivation, positive and negative. Positive motivation comes from a natural response to desire. What do you desire from exercise? Is it the way it makes you look and feel, or could it be the increased strength and stability it will give you during your next skiing vacation, for example? You want to exercise because of the desired outcome.

Negative motivation is derived, in this context, from the result of not exercising. For example, "I will put on weight if I do not exercise" or "I must exercise tonight, because if I miss any more sessions I will

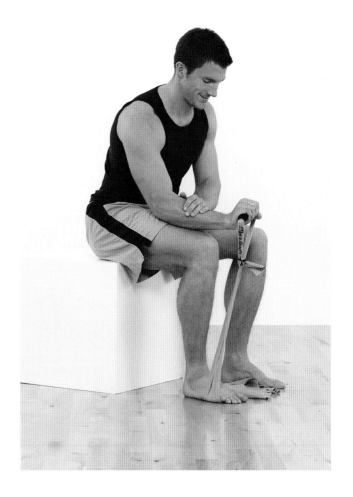

motivation

never become fitter." Eventually, negative motivation creates stress. This can cause people to stop exercising, because of the mind's resistance to these negative thoughts.

A way to identify negative motivation is to notice any time you use words like should, must, have to, ought to, and got to. Once you have noticed yourself using these words, change them to positive ones like "want to", "feel like", and "would like to." It creates less internal resistance from your mind.

Find the positive good in the reasons for exercising correctly and consistently. Notice any negative motivation and transform it into positive, letting your desire for that positive good be your primary motivation.

By reading this book, you will understand the basic fundamentals of exercise—warming-up, stretching, warming-down, etc—and learn that exercising within your chosen zones will assist you in attaining your desired outcome. Results come through consistency, and this is why you will want to set time aside during your week to exercise. Remember that any time you say, "I should", you can change this to, "I want to", and "I must" can become, "I will." In doing so, you will notice an elevation of the stress involved and enjoy being empowered to motivate yourself toward your desired result.

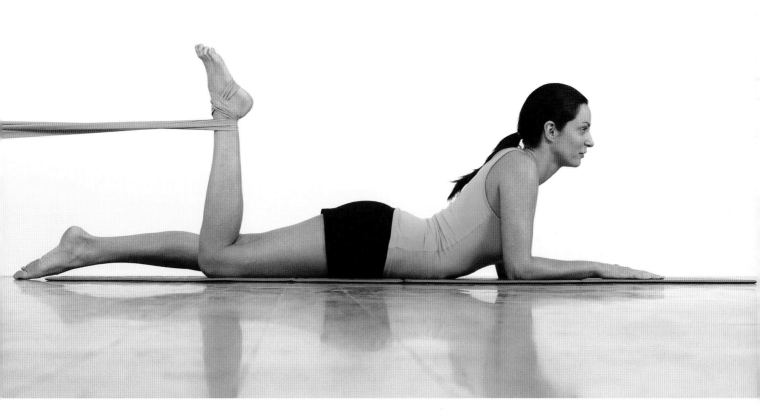

When reading and looking at an exercise or stretch, visualize yourself doing the resistance band exercise before you physically do it. There are several reasons for visualizing, and one of them is to enable you to develop your own set of exercises in time to come. As mentioned earlier, the possibilities for the use of resistance bands in exercise and sport development are limited only by your imagination. This visualization technique will enable you to practice the exercise correctly, so you will maximize the benefit from the exercises and reduce the likelihood of improper resistance band technique and resulting injury.

All top sports people visualize before executing the technique for real. Top golfers, for example, never take a swing, either in practice or in a tournament, without having first visualized the stroke, and when visualizing, they hit the shot perfectly, every time. When you visualize any form of exercise, ensure your technique is perfect.

The reason for this is that when we visualize, picturing with feeling and with all our senses active in this visualization, our brain sends minute signals to the muscles involved in the action we are "seeing." The neurological pathways are being made, even though we are not actually doing the exercise. A great example many of us have experienced is when we are dreaming. Our body may twitch and seem to move involuntarily in reaction to what we are dreaming. The brain's signals are as if the event were real—and for the muscles, it is real, there is no difference.

There is an important link between visualization and motivation. Using negative motivation, stating what you do not want, creates a visual image of what you do not want. This image draws you farther toward what you do not want to happen. An example of this negative draw is: "I do not want to lose my balance."

Did you think of losing your balance, even though you were trying not to? Using positive motivation leads us toward what we want, our desired outcome. A positive approach to the previous example would be: "I will maintain my balance."

By reading the exercise directions and observing the images of that exercise, picture yourself doing the exercise and doing it perfectly and positively. You should be associated with the visualization. That means imagining everything as if you are both seeing and feeling—that is, imagine how the motion of the exercise acts on your muscles. Add sounds and other sensory cues that are associated with the event, such as the noise of the band stretching, even the smell of the band. Correct yourself if you notice that you are using statements such as: "Don't bend my back." Correct this to: "Keep my back straight." By doing so, and by executing the visualized technique perfectly, you are setting yourself up for success. This will help you with your balance and your posture while using the resistance band. This is your body, and you can maximize its control and function. Have the motivation to incorporate visualization into your learning of the exercises. Incorporate this into your chosen sport.

visualization

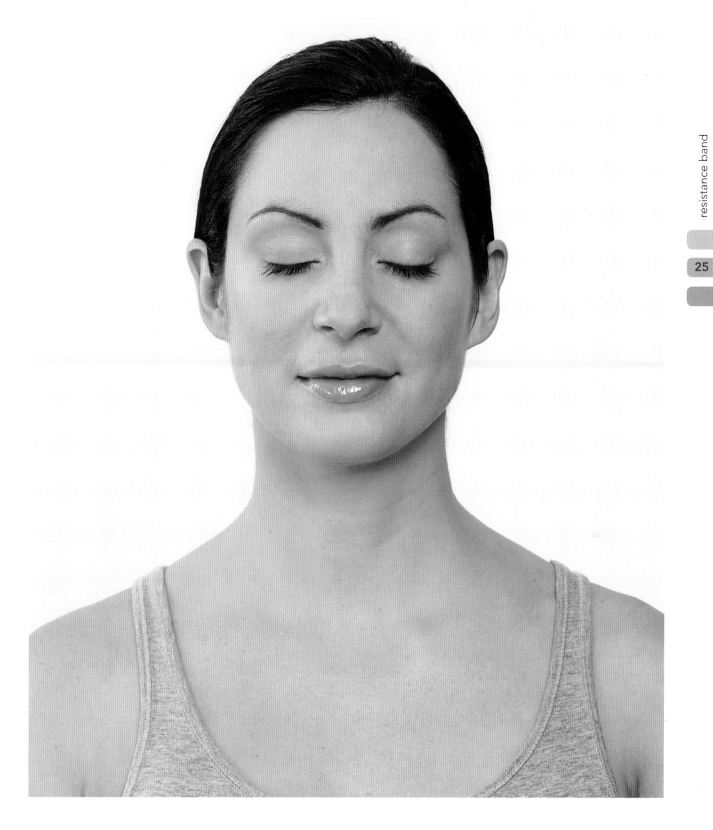

Now that you know all about
resistance bands and your body,
it is time to bring it together.

A resistance band is wonderfully simple, yet highly
effective. Because of its compact nature, you will
be able to exercise just about anywhere. You will
probably have thought of the many benefits and
possibilities the resistance band and its exercises
will bring you, especially if you travel often, or are
required to be at home for much of the time. The
key is consistency.

Having read the section on basic anatomy, you now
have an understanding of the different body types
and how assorted resistance exercises affect them.
So what's next?

• Decide what your goals are if you have not done
so already. What is your reason for exercising with
resistance bands?

• Look at the body-type section and decide which
of the four body types described best matches your
own. Be honest with yourself and reassess at any time
to ensure you are giving yourself the best type of
workout for your needs.

• Work out your maximum heart rate as shown,
and practice finding and taking your own pulse. It
soon becomes quite easy to calculate your beats
per minute. Remember your maximum heart rate,
because you will be monitoring your heart's progress
as you exercise within the zones, and do not exceed
this maximum.

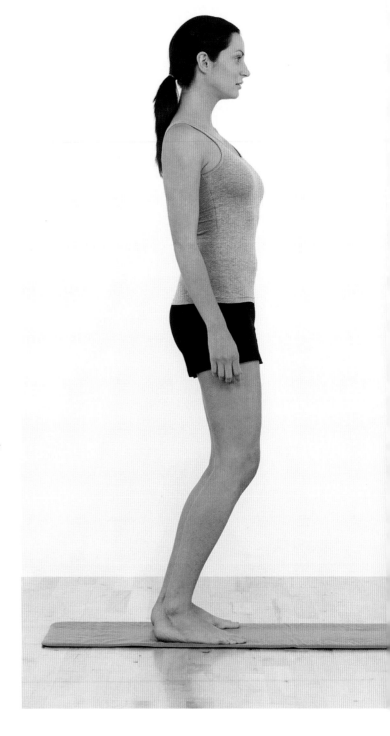

how to use this book

• Knowing why you want to exercise is the key to motivating yourself and being successful. Do practice your awareness and use of motivational words. Notice the words you use to yourself and to others. Are you positively or negatively motivated? Use the simple but truly effective method you have learned for altering and maintaining your motivation.

• The chapters following this introduction will show you how to stretch and exercise with the resistance band, and offer you sample exercise charts. Once you have read through the exercises and the charts, you will be able to decide upon the right type of exercises for you and the resistance intensity with which to perform them.

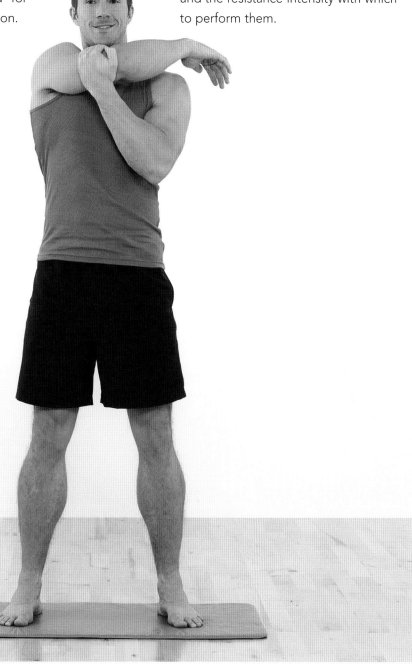

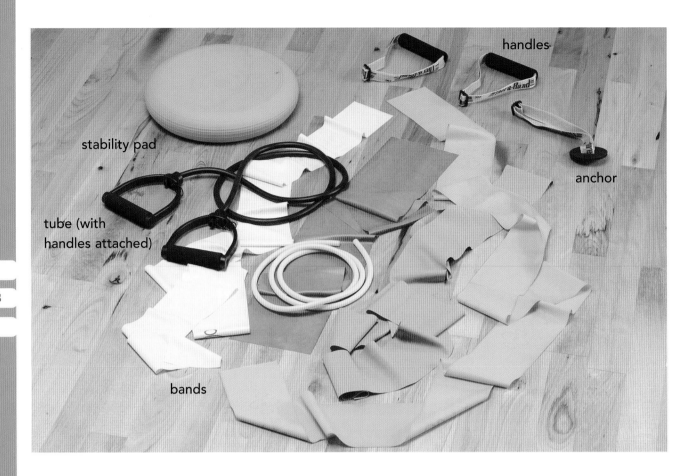

handles

stability pad

tube (with
handles attached)

anchor

bands

Resistance bands, tubes, and accessories

There are many elastic band resistance products on the market, most developed from the two basic options of the resistance band and the resistance tube. The two do not differ in principle, concept, or mechanics. Choosing between a band and a tube is a matter of personal preference. Bands tend to be favored because they can be simply wrapped about the hand or body part, without having to be attached to a fixed object. Tubes tend to be preferred for upper body exercises and bands for lower. Tubes and bands are also produced in closed loops and in various dimensions.

Both bands and tubing come in different lengths and many resistance levels. The bands or tubes are color-coded according to their resistance levels. Generally, both the color and resistance of the band and tube start light and progress through to darker colors, representing increased resistance. Products

are generally made from Latex, although Latex-free resistance products are available for those with a Latex allergy.

It is important to attach the end of the band securely to prevent injury. There are numerous useful accessories available to enhance your resistance training, such as door anchors and handles. These provide additional safety and comfort when training.

The door anchor is a flat nylon strap with a buckled loop at one end to attach the resistance band or tube and a firm foam pad at the other. Simply position the anchor's flat nylon strap by the door frame with the foam pad positioned on the opposite side of the door frame, then close the door and lock it. This will ensure that the resistance band or tube can be held in position firmly and safely when you apply force to it when exercising.

Safety

- Get approval from your health adviser before undertaking resistance exercises, especially if you have musculoskeletal problems.

- Use Latex-free products if you have a Latex allergy.

- Ensure the band is secured to your chosen anchor point. If using a door as an anchor point, make sure it is securely closed and locked to prevent sudden opening.

- Protect the resistance band from jewelry, sharp objects, and fingernails.

- Note that bands degrade if left out in direct sunlight and extremes of temperature.

- Never point a band under tension toward your face.

- Follow the pre- and post-exercise guidelines explained in this book. Ensure you first warm up and then stretch before exercising, and warm down when you have completed your workout.

- Maintain correct posture when exercising.

- If you feel pain during an exercise, stop immediately. Reassess to ensure that you are doing the exercise correctly and that you have not skipped your pre-exercise warm-up and stretching phase. Reduce the tension used during that exercise. If pain persists, consult your health professional.

- If your heart rate increases faster and is unusually high during warm-up and/or during exercise, stop exercising. It is an indication that you are tired and your immune system could be fighting off the beginnings of an illness. If symptoms persist, visit your health care professional.

Posture and form

It is important to maintain good posture when exercising. This will reduce the chances of injury and give you maximum benefit from each exercise. The visualization technique will assist you to maintain proper posture and form throughout the exercises.

When standing, have your feet shoulder-width apart, unless otherwise stated, with soft knees (not locked). Keep your lower back and neck in a neutral position, with your shoulders back and down. Make sure you do not twist or arch your back to complete an exercise. Stabilize your torso and improve your core stability by strengthening your abdominal and lower back muscles when exercising. Activate your core muscles by sucking in your stomach while exhaling, and, when you feel your stomach muscles contract, lock them into this contracted position and continue to breathe normally. Activating your core muscles will give you maximum benefit when exercising and improve your results.

The correct motion of the exercise is a combination of your posture and technique or form. When muscles become tired, there is a tendency to "cheat" by employing different muscle groups to assist, which can lead to injury. Ensure smooth and controlled extensions and contractions during each exercise and maintain your breathing.

BREATHING

Never hold your breath during any part of the exercise, as this can lead to light-headedness or even fainting. Exhale slowly as you apply tension and inhale through the return phase.

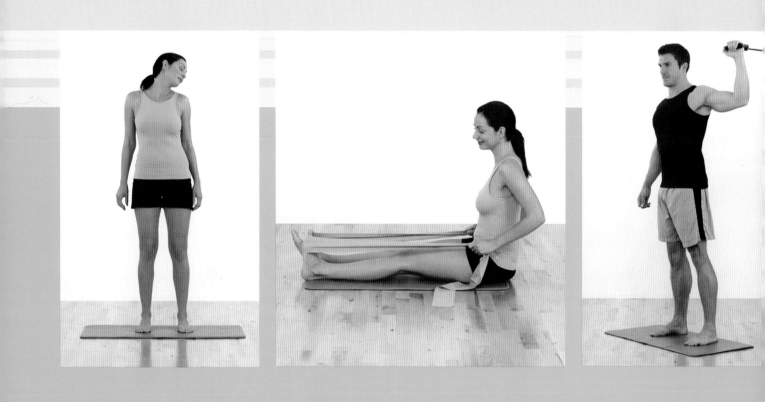

2

warm-up and stretching

In this chapter, you will learn why it is essential to warm-up and stretch and to include a proper warm-down after you exercise. The benefits of these will be explained, as well as how these elements will help you toward your desired goal.

The warm-up increases your body temperature and the temperature deep within your muscles. Warming up raises your heart rate gradually, preparing you both physically and mentally for your resistance band exercises to come.

Stretching should commence only after you have warmed up. Stretching will do much more than just increase your flexibility, and in this chapter you will learn why it is so important.

Warming down after exercise is equally important, and you will receive the full benefits of your exercise only if you have cooled down properly.

You will gain maximum benefit from resistance band exercise if you follow the fundamental phases of exercise—warm-up, stretch, exercise, and warm-down.

A general warm-up will prepare both your body and mind for exercise. It begins with gentle joint rotation. Start either from your fingers and work your way down, or from your toes and work your way up. These gentle rotations, in both clockwise and counterclockwise directions, facilitate the joints to release synovial fluid, a lubricant that increases the joint's mobility and function when called upon during exercise.

JOINT ROTATION

fingers and knuckles • wrists • elbows • shoulders • neck • trunk/waist • hips • legs • knees • ankles • toes

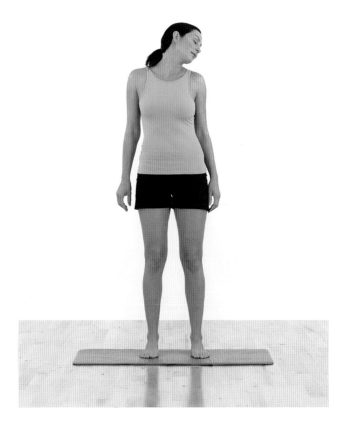

After performing the joint rotations, you should engage in light aerobic activity such as jogging on the spot, light skipping (jump rope), stationary cycling, or easy rowing. It should be of sufficient duration and intensity to raise your heart rate to about 50–60% of your maximum heart rate without developing fatigue. It should take between 5 and 15 minutes for your body to feel loose and break into a steady sweat, raising your core body temperature and getting your blood flowing. Increased blood flow in your muscles improves muscle performance and flexibility and reduces the likelihood of injury.

No more than 10 minutes should elapse between completing your warm-up and performing the resistance band exercises.

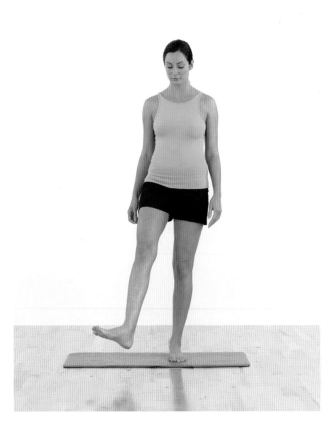

Once warmed up, begin to stretch. Engage in some slow, relaxed, static stretching, taking between 4 and 7 minutes depending upon your age and flexibility. Start with your back, followed by your upper body and lower body, stretching all your major muscle groups.

Stretching increases your flexibility, which helps to increase your body tone and your ability to avoid injury, and increases your range of motion. Never bounce up and down or stretch until you feel pain. Correct static stretches target the muscle and connecting tissues passively. Stretch until you feel a mild tension, then relax by exhaling a deep breath, then breathe normally as you maintain the stretch. This method enables the muscles to lengthen to their greatest possible extent.

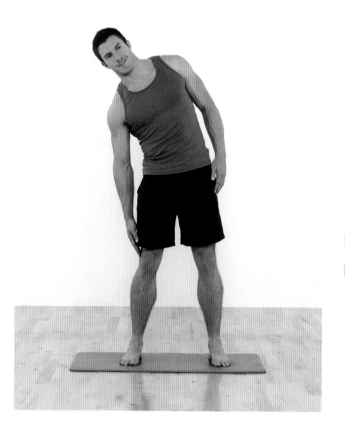

PNF STRETCHING

One of the most effective methods of stretching is called proprioceptive neuromuscular facilitation (PNF). You can facilitate a PNF stretch utilizing the resistance band.

• Take the joint to the end of its range of motion, stretching until you feel a mild tension, then relax with an exhalation of a deep breath. Now breathe normally, maintaining the stretch.

• Utilizing the resistance band, apply mild force (10–20%) muscle pressure against the band in the opposite direction to your stretch for 6 seconds, then relax your resistance, enabling the band's tension to stretch your muscle farther to its new lengthened position for another 10–20 seconds. Let the resistance band ease the muscle gently into this lengthened position without any input from you, except that of relaxing.

• Again apply 10–20% muscle pressure against the band in the opposite direction to your stretch for 6 seconds, then again relax your resistance, enabling the band's tension to stretch your muscle farther to its new lengthened position. Remain in this new position for 10–20 seconds to set your muscle's new length. Repeat this PNF stretching process 3–4 times.

Upper trapezius PNF stretch

Imagine the movement of bringing your left shoulder and your left ear close together by shrugging your left shoulder and tilting your head to the right. Take a moment, now, to visualize this movement, ending with a deep breath and exhaling, releasing any tension the image created, and then relax.

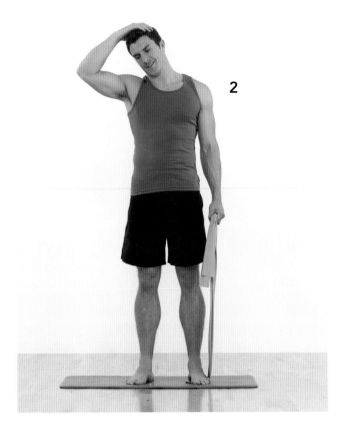

1 Stand with your left foot in the middle of a doubled band. Clasp the ends of the band in your left hand, ensuring there is tension in the band when your left arm is fully extended downward at your side.

2 Tilt your head to the right and look downward, using your right hand to hold your head gently in this position.

3 Keeping your left arm straight, shrug your left shoulder upward, applying mild force (10–20%) on the band. At the same time, use your right hand to resist gently the movement of your head. The rest of your spine remains straight. Hold this position for 6 seconds, breathing naturally throughout.

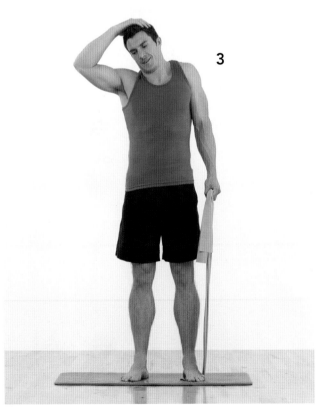

4 Taking a deep breath, exhale and gently relax both your head and shoulder, enabling the resistance band to release your shoulder downward, with your right hand maintaining your head tilted toward the right. This will lengthen your upper left trapezius.

5 Breathing normally, hold this position for 10–15 seconds.

6 Repeat the stretch 3–4 times on the left side, then repeat the exercise on the right side.

Pectoralis major

Overworking the chest area can shorten the pectoralis major muscles, restricting your ability to lift your arms above your head. It also causes forward or medial rotation of the shoulder, so that when you swing your arms as you walk, your palms face backward and not to your sides.

1 Secure a doubled resistance band at shoulder height to a fixed object, such as a locked door, using a resistance band anchor.

2 Clasping the band in your left hand, stand with your back to the anchor point and your left elbow and shoulder both at 90-degree angles, as if taking an oath. The band's tension should be enough to stretch the front part of your shoulder gently.

3 Maintaining your elbow position, gently rotate your shoulder inward with 10–20% force against the resistance band. Hold this static position, breathing normally throughout, for 6 seconds.

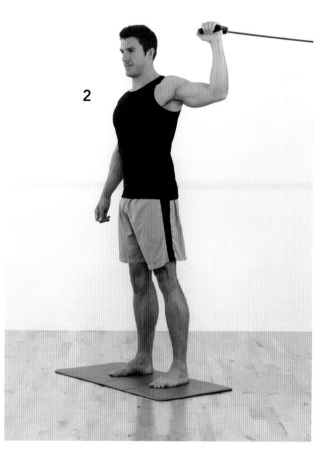

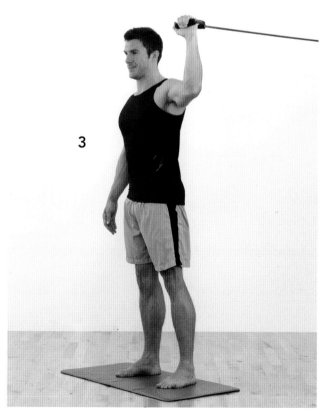

4 Take a deep breath, then relax as you exhale slowly. Let the band return your shoulder to just beyond your start position. Notice the reduction in tension within the pectoralis major muscle as you exhale and relax, increasing the muscle's length.

5 Breathing normally, hold this position for 10–15 seconds.

6 Repeat the stretch 3–4 times, then repeat the exercise on the right side.

Quadriceps

The quadriceps are the group of four muscles located to the front of each thigh. Ensuring that these muscles are flexible can assist the correct movement of your knees when walking or running, and can help relieve lower back pain.

1 Lie on your front with the resistance band looped around your right shin or foot and your right knee bent to around a 90-degree angle.

2 With the resistance band stretching from your foot passing over your right shoulder, hold the ends of the band in both hands with your arms stretched out in front of you. Ensure you are in a stable and comfortable position on the floor. Maintain enough tension in the resistance band so that it stretches your quadriceps until you feel a mild tension.

3 Start to apply 10–20% of your quadriceps' strength, opposing the pull of the resistance band by initiating the straightening of your right knee. Your lower leg will move slightly away from your body as the resistance band absorbs your force, then remain in a static position, with the force of the band equal to that of your quadriceps. Hold this position for 6 seconds, breathing naturally throughout.

4 Taking a deep breath, exhale and gently relax the quadriceps, letting the resistance band return your knee to the start position. Notice your knee has bent a little farther, which is normal because the stretch lengthens the quadriceps. Breathing normally, hold this position for 10–20 seconds.

5 Repeat the stretch 3–4 times, then repeat the exercise on the left side.

2

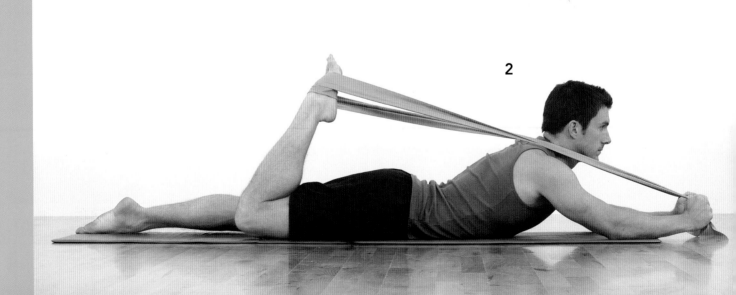

Hamstrings

The hamstrings are the group of three muscles located at the rear of each thigh. Ensuring these powerful muscles are flexible can assist in preventing knee pain and can help relieve lower back pain.

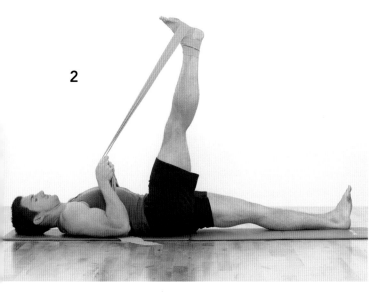

1 Lie on your back with both legs flat and the resistance band looped under your right foot. Hold the ends of the band in both hands.

2 Keeping your leg straight, use the band to lift your right leg upward, until you feel a mild tension in your hamstrings.

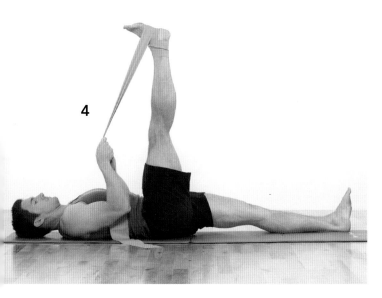

3 Push the right leg downward toward the floor with 10–20% force against the resistance band, keeping your knee straight. You will probably need to pull with your hands to increase the amount of force being applied by the band to equal the downward movement of your leg. Hold this position for 6 seconds, breathing normally.

4 With a deep breath, exhale and relax your hamstrings, letting the resistance band pull your leg gently back toward and beyond your extended starting position. Notice that your hamstrings will have lengthened. Ensure that your back remains flat on the floor and that you are not lifting your hips or your left leg off the floor. Hold this relaxed stretched position for 10–20 seconds.

5 Repeat the stretch 3–4 times, then repeat the exercise on the left side.

THINK POSITIVELY

Remember your desired outcome and why it is important to stretch before you exercise. Alter any negative motivational thoughts, such as "I should...," to positive motivational words, such as "I want...."

Hip flexor

Imagine kneeling on your left knee, with your right foot on the floor in front of you, right knee bent to no more than 90 degrees, in the classic "will you marry me?" proposal position. Make sure your shoulders and hips are square and facing forward. This is the basic position for this stretch.

1 Secure a doubled resistance band at waist height to a solid object, such as a locked door, using a resistance band anchor.

2 Loop the band around your left thigh, just above your knee. Side-sit on a solid chair with your back to the band's attachment point. Your right buttock and thigh should be supported on the chair, with the right knee bent to 90 degrees and your right foot on the floor. Make sure your hips and pelvis are square and your back is straight. Assume the proposal position, with your left hip gently extended behind, left knee slightly bent. Let the resistance band apply mild tension to your hip and thigh muscles, adjusting your distance from the anchor point to apply sufficient tension.

3 Gently flex your left hip forward against the band's tension, 10–20% force, for 6 seconds, breathing normally. With a deep breath, exhale and relax your hip, enabling the resistance band to gently extend your hip backward beyond your starting position. Hold this relaxed stretched position for 10–20 seconds.

4 Repeat the stretch 3–4 times, then repeat the exercise on the other side.

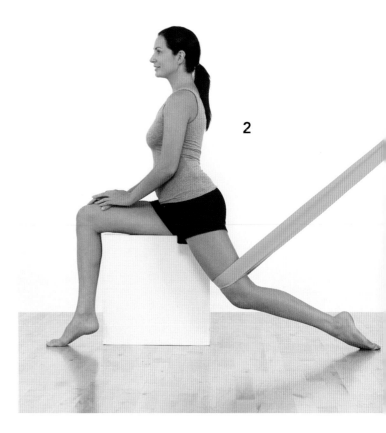

2

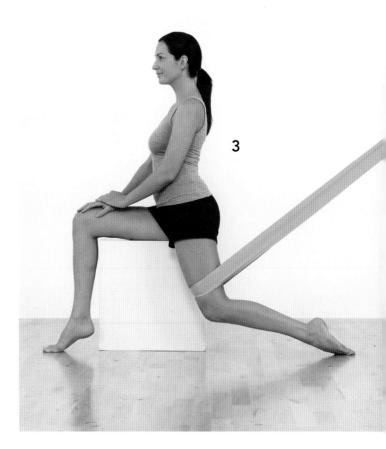

3

Gastrocnemius and soleus

The gastrocnemius and soleus muscles are located at the rear of the lower leg. Commonly known as the calf muscles, they are fundamental for running and jumping. Constant wearing of high-heeled shoes causes these muscles to shorten, which can affect posture negatively. The two muscles of the calf are stretched in similar ways except that the knee is slightly bent when stretching the soleus, whereas the gastrocnemius stretch requires your leg to be straight.

1 Sitting on the floor, with legs straight, loop the resistance band under the ball of your left foot.

2 Holding the ends of the band in both hands, stretch the band, pulling your foot backward until you feel mild tension in your calf muscles. Gently push the foot forward using 10–20% force for 6 seconds, breathing normally. You might need to pull on the band to adjust the tension at this point, to balance the force exerted by your foot.

3 Exhale deeply as you relax your calf muscles, enabling the band to pull your foot backward beyond your starting position, again until you feel mild tension. Hold this relaxed position for 10–15 seconds while breathing normally.

4 Repeat the stretch 3–4 times, then repeat the exercise on the right side.

STRETCHING

Stretching increases your flexibility, which helps to increase your body tone and your ability to avoid injury and also increases your range of motion. Never bounce up and down or stretch until you feel pain.

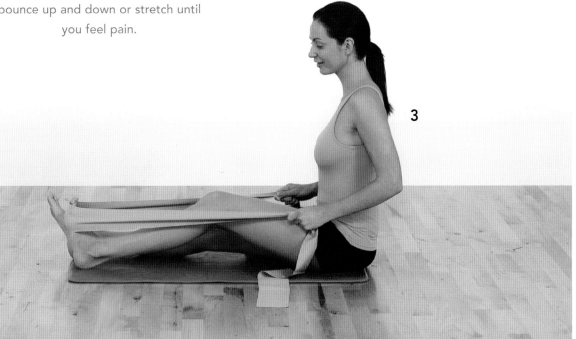

3

Piriformis

The piriformis muscles are located in the buttocks. A common problem that can be associated with tight piriformis muscles is sciatic pain, which can be reduced by stretching and lengthening these muscles.

1 Lie flat on your back with both legs extended. Keeping your left leg flat on the floor, lift and bend your right leg and lay it across your left knee. Loop the resistance band over your right thigh, just above your knee, and clasp the ends of the band in your left hand. Extend your right arm out to the side to give you extra stability, making sure your back remains in contact with the floor.

2 Gently pull the band so that your right leg crosses farther over your left knee until you feel mild tension in the right piriformis.

3 Gently pull your right thigh back toward your right side, applying 10–20% force with your right knee against the band. Breathing normally, hold the position for 6 seconds, with the force of the band equal to that of your thigh.

4 Exhale and relax your piriformis, letting the resistance band pull your right leg back to beyond the starting position until mild tension is felt. Remain relaxed by breathing normally. Maintain this position for 10–20 seconds.

5 Repeat the stretch 3–4 times, then repeat the exercise on the left side.

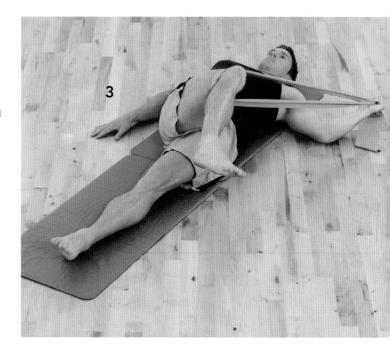

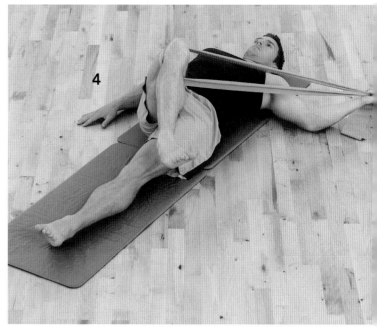

BREATHING

Never hold your breath when stretching or exercising. Exhaling after a deep breath enables you to release muscle tension in your body. This enables the muscles to relax more and therefore increases their length.

Latissimus dorsi and internal obliques

The latissimus dorsi and internal oblique muscles are heavily utilized in sports such as golf, gymnastics, swimming, rowing, and all throwing sports. This great stretch will assist you in increasing both your mobility and your range of movement.

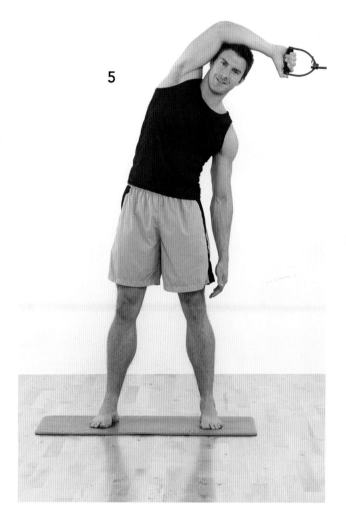

1 Securely attach the resistance band at a high level, such as at the top of a locked door, using a resistance band anchor. Stand with your left side toward the anchor point. Clasp the end of the resistance band in your right hand, with your arm raised high above your shoulder, thumb inward.

2 Move sideways away from the anchor point until the resistance band is taut. Stand with your feet close together, ensuring that you do not lean either forward or backward.

3 Keeping your right arm raised and your left foot stationary, take a side step to the right, away from the anchor point.

4 Lean your trunk toward the anchor point, enabling the resistance band to draw a mild stretch to your latissimus dorsi and internal oblique muscles on the right side.

5 Lean your trunk toward the right and gently apply 10–20% force, pulling against the resistance band. Breathing normally, hold this position for 6 seconds.

6 Exhale and relax your torso, letting the resistance band stretch you beyond your starting position until mild tension is felt. Remain relaxed by breathing normally. Maintain this position for 10–20 seconds.

7 Repeat the stretch 3–4 times, then repeat the exercise on the right side.